# Dedication

This book is dedicated to a Higher Source
who ultimately inspires those scientists,
beknown to them or not, to work hard and be
thorough in their research. These gifted men
and women have been given the incredible
healing power of PSP and alkalized water.

# Preface

Humans have survived for as many as ninety days without food, but can live only seventy-two hours without water before going into a semi-comatose state. However, drinking water saturated with inorganic minerals such as magnesium carbonate, calcium carbonate and other elements the body cannot use, may lead to a variety of unhealthy conditions. These inorganic minerals, toxic chemicals, fluoride and other contaminants can pollute, clog up and even turn tissues to stone throughout our body, causing pain, illness and even premature death. Alkalized water, nature's healing water, helps remove inorganic mineral deposits and toxins from the joints, may remove cholesterol and fat, and creates a pH balance in our body.

Nature and science are not always a marriage made in heaven. Until those in the health care profession realize the necessity of a bond between the two, millions of people will continue to suffer and die needlessly. This book is devoted to the benefits of what I believe to be the most powerful of whole food complexes and unlocking the mysteries of alkalized water, which can relieve chronic suffering. Using the healing benefits of alkalized water has been proven to help us live healthier and longer lives.

*Howard Peiper N.D.*

# Partners in Healing

# Health and Recovery with PSP and Alkalized Water

Published by WTP Publishing
(760) 902 3343

# Table of Contents

## Section 1 - ALKALIZED WATER

## Section 2 – PSP

*"Physicians think they are doing something for us by labeling what we have as a disease"*

Immanuel Kant

# Solved, The Secret Mystery of Aging!

We are programmed to get old and look old, but it doesn't have to be that way. Age and longevity are relative. Some people at age sixty-five look forty-five — others at sixty-five look eighty-five.

Nobody denies genes. Our parents have an awful lot to do with our physical and mental makeup. But we can do a great deal to improve our looks and our quality of life. Aging without quality of life is not exciting. We can make a big difference, but only if we believe that we can, and then take action.

First and most important is to know what we put in our mouth. Americans are starving to death. Yes, we are consuming larger and larger amounts of "food", getting fatter and fatter, and sicker and sicker. Nobody is enjoying this except the medical establishment. There are plenty of sick people.

Here is what's happening. We are consuming tasty foods (so-called) that have calories and produce energy but lack nutrition. Did you know that some foods have calories that produce energy but have no nutrition? This is the definition of the beautifully packaged commercial foods that we eat. In fact, this is mostly what Americans consume and we gradually starve to death.

Empty foods as described above not only do not provide nutrition, they build and accumulate as toxemia or poison in the body and in the blood. The accumulation of toxins in the body is the beginning of death. Death is the result of toxemia. Diseases and death is a common expression of toxemia.

Think, now! Disease cannot be its own cause; neither can it be its own cure — and certainly not its own prevention. We cause disease ourselves. Sickness and low quality of life go hand in hand. There is no life or vitality in antibiotics or flu shots or immunization. Life, beauty and youth are in the blood and good blood is made of good food.

Good blood, vigorous health and stamina cannot come from a subsistence on white bread,

doughnuts, pies, cakes, latte's and pretty packaged commercial foods sold at the supermar-
ket. Consider all the tens of thousands of
preparations including most so-called "health
foods" and cereals. Include all the "food" that
has been dyed or treated chemically to have a
beautiful appearance, fried, impaired and
impoverished foods, pasteurized and dead
foods.

The main causes of aging and disease are to
be found in the derangement of normal
processes of cell metabolism and cell
regeneration. The accumulation of toxins
(acidic foods) and metabolic waste products
interferes with the nourishment of the cells
and slows down cell regeneration and new cell
building. When normal metabolic processes
become deranged (due to nutritional
deficiencies, sluggish digestion and
elimination, sedentary life and overeating),
and the process of cell nourishment,
replacement and rebuilding slows down, our
body starts to grow old. Its resistance to
disease will diminish and various ills will start
to appear.

Beauty, strength, youthfulness and long life
occur because we select the right foods to put

in our bodies. It all sounds so simple, but is it? Food is not necessarily *food*.

*"There is no natural death. All deaths from so-called natural causes are merely the end point of a progressive acid saturation."*

Dr. George W. Crile

## *Acidity - The Grim Reaper!*

It is not generally known that acidity (acid foods) is the principal cause of most disease.

The accumulation of acidity (acid) in the blood and the cells is the principal cause of disease and death. Leading researchers have found that there is no natural death. All deaths from so-called natural causes are merely the end points of a progressive acid saturation (toxemia).

Most of all the foods we eat are acid forming. There are so many that we cannot name them all. Almost all processed food products are acid forming. Most bottled goods are acid forming. Fats, oils (modern cooking oils), sugars, sweets, syrups, candies, starches, baked goods, cereals, glucose, jams, and jellies are acid forming. Nearly *all* cooked, fried and baked foods are acid forming.

Almost all drugs, pills, patent medicines, drinks, tonics, wine, liquors, coffee, tea, chocolate, cocoa, and all manufactured foods are acid forming. All canned fruits almost without exception, are acid forming. Some types of canned fruit are not originally acid forming, but they become acid forming by processing; i.e., peeling, paring, cooking sweetening, preserving, or by altering and disorganizing the fruit and fruit molecules such as microwave cooking and steaming and destroying the vitamins of life. All nuts are acid forming except almonds. Most peppers and pickles are acid.

The end product of our own metabolism (catabolism) is acid forming. The products of combustion or oxidation in the body are acid forming. The dying leukocytes, dying tissues, the excreta in the bowels, the mucus, phlegm, dying bacteria, and their toxins are all acid forming. Even brain activity, thinking, worry, temper, and all sorts of unfavorable emotions result in acidity. Acidity is the father of disease.

Acid is the cause of gas generation, bloating, dullness, poor memory and low energy. So as long as we can keep the tissues nourished and keep the secretions, stomach, blood and bones alkaline, we are healthy, youthful, vigorous, efficient, lively and strong.

It is impossible to get sick so long as the human body is alkaline. It is equally impossible to keep well when the system is in an acid condition. Human alkalinity and longevity go hand in hand. Human acidity leads to disease, operations and an early funeral. An alkaline diet results in health, longevity, youth and beauty.

There is no escape from wrong choices. If we live on acid-forming foods meal after meal, year after year our body must pay the bill over and over again. Acid forming foods accumulate as toxemia. Death results from toxemia. If we must eat, we may just as well eat right. Acidity is the foundation of most of our disease, trouble, misery, pain and tears. Acidity is toxemia. Toxemia is death.

Acid in or around the nerves results in neuralgia, neuritis, sciatica, nervousness, nerve pain, headache, earache, or various nerve ailments and diseases. Acid brain matter results in inflammation of the brain, insanity, crime, violent passion, melancholia, and hundreds of symptoms of mental disease. An acid brain cannot function normally.

Acid causes arthritis, urinary ailments, heart valve problems, and kidney problems. Acidity in or around the prostate. gland causes enlargement of the prostate gland, swelling and hardening, resulting in prostate cancer or at least urinary difficulties. An acid uterus leads to female complications of the menstrual cycle, inflammation, uterine tumors, and other ailments of the generative organs.

An acid liver is a disordered liver and this may result in stubborn constipation, piles, varicosis, toxicosis, autointoxication, hepatitis, gallstones, cirrhosis of the liver, and even insanity. The acid accumulation destroys the toxilytic functions of the liver leaving autotoxins, blood toxins, bacterial toxins, and other poisons in the blood to be carried to the brain and kidneys.

Acidity in the stomach causes gastritis, heartburn and burning in the chest. Acidity causes gas generation and gas pressure upon the heart, diaphragm, spine and other organs. Gas pressure leads to dilation of the stomach until the stomach hangs like an empty, lifeless bag, resulting in falling of the stomach, bloating, colic, indigestion, cramps, and constipation. Do we see any bloated bellies in America today?

People who are waking up are taking responsibility for their own health. They are beginning to realize that the medical establishment is dependent on its human victims for its profits.

Different diets have their effects on health and disease, but acidity is the most prolific cause of disease. One chemical body type is subject to one kind of acidity, and another type is subject to another kind of acidity and gas formation.

There are many kinds of acid responses depending on the biochemistry of the individual. The most important thing to do first is to learn what is an acid food and what is an alkaline food. Human alkalinity and longevity go hand in hand.

Seldom does a doctor in America suspect that bad diet is the cause of degenerative disease. And few would suspect that the prevailing high acid diet of Americans is the root cause of early death and suffering.

The soil in America is now so poor and so poisoned with chemical fertilizers that it is nearly impossible to buy nutritious food. The only thing left for those concerned is to get the proper whole food supplement complexes (particularly organic foods) prepared and marketed by people who are knowledgeable in human health and nutrition, and to drink alkalized, filtered water.

*"Mother Nature is man's teacher. She unfolds her treasure to his search, unseals his eyes, illuminates his mind and purifies his heart.*

Dr. Bernard Jensen

# Alkalinity Conquers Death

As we grow older, it is ever more important to know the properties of food so that we make selections that are alkaline. There is always danger of acid formation and gas generation as we live longer. Poor elimination, low vitality, tissue acidity, and autointoxication all come with age because of our ignorance of acid and alkaline foods.

Health must be developed from the inside. Beauty and youthfulness are the result of a correct alkaline diet. Grace in movement, elasticity in our arteries and tendons, and joy in living are all born of a proper diet.

When we are alkalized/balanced, there is no acidity, no gas, no autotoxins, no poisons and no accumulation of toxemia. Oxygen is abundantly supplied, the brain and nerves are well nourished, and the red blood flows vigorously to all parts of the body. Then we have regained youth and enjoy a great quality of life. We can help speed up this process by drinking alkalized water as a daily routine.

Aging may be reversed by changing our diet provided we begin before we are 90 percent dead. Aging is a disease of diet, and more specifically aging is a disease of progressive acid saturation. Because we are programmed to grow old and die does not mean that it is natural. Alkalized water can help stop this deterioration!

## Acid-Forming Foods

Acid-forming foods which should be temporarily eschewed or drastically limited during the alkalization period are principally meat, fish, poultry, eggs, cheese, fats, white bread, starchy foods, cakes, pastry, candy, white sugar, and confections. These foods are not necessarily bad but should never be taken in proportions that exceed the requirement for body need.

## Alkaline Foods – (80% of diet)

| | |
|---|---|
| Celery | Apples |
| Potatoes | Bananas |
| Carrots | Citrus fruits |
| Cabbage | Beets |
| Lettuce | Cucumbers |
| Asparagus | Melons |
| Tomatoes | Raisins |
| Green Beans | Pineapples |
| Squash | Grapes |
| Parsnips | Pears |
| Almonds | Buttermilk |
| Beans | Peaches |
| Spinach | Fresh Peas |

## Acid Foods – (20% or less of diet)

| | |
|---|---|
| Meat | Rice (polished) |
| Fish | Corn (dried) |
| Poultry | Crackers |
| Cheese | Hydrogenated oil |
| Eggs | Nuts (except almonds) |
| Cereal | Spaghetti |
| Bread | White Flour |
| Refined Sugar | Chocolate |
| Candy | Coffee/Tea |
| Pastry | Alcohol |

*"The doctor of the future will give little medicine, but will interest his patients in the care of the human frame, diet, and in the cause and prevention of disease."*

Thomas A. Edison

# Dehydration - Am I Thirsty?

Did you know that 50-75 percent of Americans are chronically dehydrated and many of those individuals are drinking eight glasses of water a day?

Dehydration is a condition that occurs when a person loses more fluid than they take in. However, the problem is not just a lack of water, it is a lack of cellular water!

Every function of the body is monitored and pegged to the efficient flow of water. "Water distribution" is the only way of making sure that not only an adequate amount of water but also its transported elements (hormones, chemical messengers and nutrients) reach the more vital organs first. In turn, every organ that produces a substance to be made available to the rest of the body will monitor its own rate of production and release this substance into the "flowing water," according to constantly changing quotas set by the brain. Once the water itself reaches the "drier" areas it also exercises its many other vital physical and chemical regulatory actions.

Water intake and its priority distribution achieve paramount importance. The regulating neurotransmitter systems (histamine and its subordinate agents) become increasingly active during the regulation of water requirements of the body.

## Water intake and Thirst Sensations

There are basically three stages to water regulation of the body in the different phases of life. One: the stage of life of a fetus in the uterus of the mother. Interestingly when the very first indicator for water needs of the fetus appear the mother seems to get morning sickness during the early phase of pregnancy. Two: the phase of growth to adulthood. Three: the phase of growth to the demise of the person. Because of a gradually failing thirst sensation our body becomes chronically and increasingly dehydrated, starting from the early adult stage.

With increase in age the water content of the cells of the body decrease to the point that the ratio of the volume of body water inside the cells to that which is outside the cells, changes from 1.2 to 0.9. This is a drastic change. Since the "water" we drink provides the cell function and its volume requirements, the decrease in our daily water intake affects the efficiency of cell activity. It is the reason for the loss of water volume held inside the cells of the body. As a result, chronic dehydration causes symptoms that mimic disease, especially when we don't recognize the fact that we are dehydrated.

The human body can become dehydrated even when abundant water is readily available. We seem to lose our thirst sensation and the critical perception of needing water. Not recognizing our water need we become gradually, increasingly, and chronically dehydrated with progress in age. Further confusion lies in the idea that when we're thirsty, many of us often substitute tea, coffee, or alcohol-containing beverages.

The "dry mouth" is the very last sign of dehy-dration. The body can suffer from dehydration even when the mouth may be fairly moist. Still worse, in the elderly the mouth can be seen to be obviously dry and yet thirst may not be acknowledged and satisfied.

The best times to drink water are: one glass half-hour before eating food -- breakfast, lunch, and dinner -- and the same amount two hours or more after each meal. This is the very minimum amount of water our body needs. If needed, two more glasses of water should be taken around the heaviest meal or before going to bed.

Do not forget that at each phase of life, our body is the product of time-operated series of chemical interactions. It is very possible to reverse some reactions. We need not to "drown" ourselves in water. The cells of the body are like sponges; it takes some time before they become better hydrated. Also do not forget that some of them make their membranes less permissive of water diffusion, in or out.

## Color of Urine

The normal color of urine should not be dark. It should ideally be almost colorless to light yellow. If it begins to become dark yellow, or even orange in color, we are becoming dehydrated. It means the kidneys are working hard to get rid of toxins in the body in very concentrated urine. That is why urine becomes darker in color. Dark color urine is a *good* sign of dehydration.

*"The natural healing force within us is the greatest force in getting well."*

Hippocrates, Father of Medicine

# pH and Cellular Health

The abbreviation pH stands for the power of hydrogen. A pH test using a piece of litmus paper actually measures the concentration of positively charged hydrogen ions in our body. Ions are electrically charged atoms or groups of atoms that together make up the electrical "juice" or current our body uses to communicate. The more positively-charged hydrogen ions are present; the more acidity is present. The fewer hydrogen ions are present, the less acidity. The total pH scale ranges from one to fourteen, with seven considered neutral. Anything below seven is considerate acidic and anything above seven is considered alkaline.

A healthy body functions best when it is slightly alkaline. Deviations in the blood above or below a pH range of 7.30-7.45 can signal potentially serious and dangerous symptoms of diseases. When our cell and tissue pH levels deviate from a healthy range (7.2-7.5) into an acidic state (below 7.0), the acid wastes normally back up, as in a clogged sewage system.

The pH of our blood, tissues, and bodily fluids affects the state of our cellular health and internal cleanliness. When our pH levels are in proper balance, we will experience a high degree of health and wellbeing. Every metabolic and organ/system function depends entirely on our delicately balanced pH, including all regulatory mechanisms such as digestion, metabolism, respiration, hormone release, neurotransmitter release, and immunity.

It is important to understand that the pH of our blood is critical to our lives, and to our very survival. The pH of blood has a very small degree of tolerance for variation. Our body does everything in its power to keep the pH of our blood within this neutral range, between 7.30-7.45, including pulling alkalizing minerals such as calcium out our bones and other body stores, if necessary.

If the body is overwhelmed by excess acids from poor diet or over-exposure to chemical and environmental toxins, built-in compensating mechanisms go into effect in an attempt to neutralize and excrete acidic toxins from the blood, cells, lymph, and tissue fluids. There are eight internal buffering systems the body uses to neutralize acids and balance pH. If these eight neutralizing mechanisms become overwhelmed and cannot function adequately, the excess acids will severely compromise cellular integrity and function, eventually causing a complete metabolic and system breakdown where serious health problems such as cancer may manifest.

We live and die at the cellular level. All the cells (billions of them) that make up the human body are slightly alkaline and must maintain alkalinity in order to function and remain healthy and alive. However, their cellular activity creates acid and this acid is what gives the cell energy and function. As each alkaline cell performs its task of respiration it secretes metabolic wastes, and these end products of cellular metabolism are acid in nature.

Although these wastes are used for energy and function, they must not be allowed to build up. One example of this is the often painful lactic acid which is created through exercise. The body will go to any lengths to neutralize and detoxify these acids before they act as poisons in and around the cell, ultimately changing the environment of the cell. Most people and clinical practitioners believe the immune system is the body's first line of defense, but actually it is not. It is very important, but more like a very sophisticated clean-up service. We must instead look at the importance of pH balance as the first and major line of defense against sickness and disease and for health and vitality.

If we were to ask, "what is killing us," the answer might be "acidosis". Research has shown that an acidic, anaerobic (lacking oxygen) body environment encourages the breeding of fungus, mold, bacteria, and viruses. A state of acidosis is simply the lack of oxygen and available calcium, which the body uses to maintain its alkaline balance. Calcium makes up 1.5 percent of our body weight. It is literally the human glue that holds the body together. A calcium ion can hold onto six other molecules while it grabs onto one molecule of water. No other ion can do this. And it does this by taking a chain of nutrients into the cell and then leaves it to get more nutrients.

The biggest problem scientists have found is that over time the human body becomes depleted of calcium. A compound called mono-ortho-calcium phosphate is the chemical buffer for the blood. This buffer maintains the alkaline level (or the lack of acidity) in our blood. Without it we would die. If the acidity level in our blood changes even slightly we die immediately. But in order to supply enough calcium for buffering we must have enough calcium being absorbed from our diet or our body will simply extract the needed calcium from our bones and teeth.

The more acidic we become, the harder it is for oxygen to be present. Therefore, our biological terrain (inside our body) also becomes anaerobic. Without adequate oxygenation unfriendly bacteria, molds, viruses, and fungus can live and prosper. Our cells cannot carry on their life-giving functions in an efficient manner because our biological chemical reactions need oxygen.

The human body is very intelligent. As we become more and more acidic the body starts to set up defense mechanisms to keep the damaging acid from entering our vital organs. Acid gets stored in fat cells. If the acid does come into contact with an organ, the acid has a chance literally to eat holes in the tissue. This may cause cells to mutate. The oxygen level drops in this acidic environment and calcium begins to be depleted. So as a defense mechanism our body may actually make fat to protect us from our overly acidic self. Those fat cells and cellulite deposits may actually be packing up the acid and trying to keep it a safe distance from our organs. The fat may be saving our vital organs from damage. Many people have found that a return to health helps them to lose the excess fat.

Osteoporosis is very confusing for many people. Most people think they can eliminate it by increasing their consumption of milk and dairy products. But in countries where the consumption of dairy products is low the instances of osteoporosis is rare. Osteoporosis is an acidosis problem. As the body becomes more acidic, to protect against the event of heart attack, stroke, illness, or even cancer, the body attempts to remain healthy. So, it steals calcium from the bones, teeth, and tissue. As bone mass becomes depleted, this is what we call osteoporosis. As we saturate the body with calcium this brings the alkaline pH up (and drops the acid levels).

One of the first warning signs of being too acidic is the appearance of calcium deposits. A little known fact is that there has never been a scientifically proven association between calcium deposits in the body and nutritional calcium. In fact, quite the opposite is found in the results of testing calcium deposits of the body. Calcium deposits come not from dietary calcium but from the structural calcium of our bones and teeth!

When the body is overwhelmed by acidosis-toxicity, mechanisms are triggered to help neutralize the buildup of poisonous acids in order to maintain a healthy, alkaline pH. Alkaline solutions (pH over 7.0) tend to absorb oxygen, while acids (pH under 7.0) tend to expel oxygen. For example, a mild alkali can absorb over 100 times as much oxygen as a mild acid. So it's a two-way street. The more acid in the body, the less ability the body fluids have to absorb oxygen. This is the classic *spiral downward* into disease. The more oxygen in the body, the more ability its fluid has to absorb oxygen. This is the *upward spiral* of health.

The first thing the body does to fight acidity is take in more oxygen the only way it knows how - through breathing harder so that it can push more $CO_2$ (carbonic Dioxide) out of the lungs and make room for more oxygen in the blood. Almost everyone wants more energy. How many people get winded and pant easily with a minimum of effort expended. That's low oxygen and over-acid condition plainly expressing itself when there isn't enough oxygen.

In low-oxygen cellular environments, excess carbon dioxide (carbonic acid) and lactic acid collect, so the body oxygen and intra-cellular amino acids are used up trying to buffer these acids. Lymph and saliva try to neutralize and dilute the acids, but they each thicken more as we dehydrate-thereby lowering their efficiency.

Next, our high pH electrolytes (calcium, magnesium, sodium, and potassium) are used up binding salt acids. Then our skin, urinary tract, colon and respiratory system become overloaded trying to filter them out. Then blood plasma changes while loading with bicarbonate in an attempt to neutralize the increasing acidity. If the low oxygen and minerals and water conditions persist and no change in oxygen levels, diet, or elimination are forth-coming, then the bones, teeth, joints and muscles will be robbed of their calcium, magnesium, sodium, and potassium reserves. This causes severe mineral deficiency. And, when all this fails (because the acidic mucoid sludge continues to block everything and pile up) then the body pushes the excess acids and toxins away from the core and out to be stored in the peripheral vital areas of the skin and extremities.

## Diseases Related Emergency Peripheral Toxin Storage

- Acid and toxins in the wrist: carpal tunnel syndrome

- Acid and toxins in the knees: osteoarthritis

- Acid and toxins in the feet and toes: gout

- Acid and toxins in the skin: dermatitis and eczema

- Acid and toxins in the joints: rheumatoid arthritis

- Acid and toxins in the tissue: fibromyalgia, chronic fatigue, and degenerative disease, etc., etc.

- Acid and toxins in the vital organs: cancer, heart disease and serious arthritis.

## The Intelligence of Cell Health

Our genetic script runs the liver's molecular machinery to store and release sugar molecules, synthesize cholesterol, detoxify the blood, secret bile and digest hemoglobin pigment. This works in tandem with the colon cells that are simultaneously fermenting aerobic bacteria, absorbing fluid, and moving your breakfast through the intestinal tract.

Each of our molecules is a delicate instrument producing a flurry of electro-chemical impulses organized by ranks of molecular switches. These turn on and off at certain intervals when necessary. A healthy body depends upon a high level of negative electromagnetic charge on tissue cells' surfaces. Acidity generates a positive charge that dampens out these electrical fields, affecting cellular communication. Unless a treatment actually removes acid toxins from the body and increases oxygen, water, and nutrients, the cure at best will only be temporary. Otherwise, the disease is driven deeper into a chronic state. The only way to properly treat disease conditions is to alkalize the pH which will dispose acids from our cells, tissues, and organs.

*"The body and mind are so closely connected that not even a single word or thought can come into existence without being reflected in the personality and health of the individual."*

John Prentiss

# Weight Gain, High Blood Pressure and Cholesterol

The central control system in the brain happens to recognize the low energy levels available for its functions. The sensations of thirst or hunger also stems from low, ready to access energy levels. To mobilize energy from that which is stored in the fat we need our hormonal release mechanisms. This process takes a while longer than the urgent needs of the brain. The front of the brain either gets energy from "hydroelectricity" or from sugar in blood circulation. Its functional needs for hydroelectricity are more urgent — not only the energy formation from water, but also its transport system within the microstream flow system that depends on more water.

The sensation of thirst and hunger are generated simultaneously to indicate the brain's needs. We do not recognize the sensation of thirst and assume "both indicators" to be the urge to eat. We eat food even when the body needs to receive water. Drinking water before eating food helps to separate the two sensations. Therefore, we are able to eat less.

High blood pressure (essential hypertension) is the result of an adaptive process to a gross body water deficiency. When we do not drink enough water to serve all the needs of the body some cells become dehydrated and lose some of their water to the circulation. Capillary beds in some areas will have to close so that some of the slack in capacity is adjusted for. In water shortage and body drought, 66 percent is lost from water held in the cells, 27 percent is taken from water volume held outside the cells, and 7 percent is taken from blood volume. The blood cells then close lumen (void space just inside the cell wall) to compensate for the water loss, causing hypertension. Therefore, the major cause for blood volume loss is the loss of body water or its undersupply through the loss of thirst sensation — and when we lose thirst sensation (or do not recognize signals of hydration) and drink less water than the daily requirement, the shutting down of some

31

vascular beds is the *only* natural alternative to keep the rest of the blood vessels full.

When diuretics are administered to remove excess water, the body becomes more dehydrated. The "dry mouth" from dehydration is reached and some water is taken to compensate. Diuretics cannot solve the problem of water retention because it is *caused* by dehydration.

Higher blood cholesterol is a sign that the cells of the body have developed a defense mechanism against the osmotic force of the blood that keeps drawing water out through the cell membranes to maintain normal cell function. Cholesterol production in the cell membrane is a part of the cell survival system. It is a necessary substance. Its excess denotes dehydration.

In a well-hydrated cell membrane, water is the adhesive material that also diffuses through the hydrocarbon "bricks". The bilayer is separated and the space is used as a "waterway" for enzyme activity. In a dehydrated cell membrane cholesterol is manufactured to stick the "bricks" together and also prevents further loss of water from inside the cell. If we drink water before we eat food, the battle against cholesterol formation in the blood can be won.

# Rheumatoid Arthritis Pain

Over 60 million Americans suffer from some form of arthritis, 30 million people suffer from low back pain, millions suffer from arthritic neck pains, and over 300,000 children are affected by the juvenile form of arthritis. Once any of these conditions establishes in an individual it becomes a sentence to suffering.

Rheumatoid arthritic joints and their pain are to be viewed as indicators of water deficiency in the affected joint cartilage surfaces. Arthritis pain is another of the regional thirst signals of the body.

The cartilage surfaces of bones in a joint contain much water. The lubricating property of this "held water" is utilized in the cartilage allowing the two opposing surfaces to freely glide over one another during joint movement.

The bone cells are immersed in calcium deposits and the cartilage cells are immersed in a matrix containing much water. As the cartilage surfaces glide over one another, some exposed cells die and peel away. New cells take their place from the growing ends that are attached to the bone surfaces on the two sides. In a well-hydrated cartilage, the rate of friction damage is minimal. In a dehydrated cartilage, the rate of "abrasive" damage is increased.

## Low Back Pain

Spinal joints, intervertebral joints and their disc structures, are depended on different hydraulic properties of water stored in the disc core, as well as in the end plate cartilage covering the flat surfaces of the spinal vertebrae. In spinal vertebral joints water is not only a lubricant for the contact surfaces, it is held in the disc core within the intervertebral space and supports the compression weight of the upper body.

Seventy-five percent of the weight of the upper part of the body is supported by water volume that is stored in the disc core and twenty-five percent is supported by the fibrous material around the disc. The principle in the design of *all* joints is for water to act as a lubricating agent, as well as to bear the force produced by weight, or tension produced by muscle action on the joint. Once dehydration sets in, all parts of the body begin to suffer. The intervertebral discs and their joints are the first in line. The 5$^{th}$ lumbar disc is affected in ninety-six percent of cases.

*We are enslaved by anything we do not consciously see. We are freed by conscious perception.*

Vernon Howard

# Cellular Oxygen Deficiency and Cancer

One of the most provocative theories regarding the cause of cancer was originally put forth by Nobel laureate Dr. Otto Warburg. He was a German biochemist who won the Nobel Prize in 1931 for discovering that oxygen deficiency and cell fermentation are part of the cancer process.

According to Dr. Warburg's theory, when cells are deprived of oxygen they can revert to their "primitive" state and enter into glucose reactions, deriving energy not from oxygen as normal plant and animal cells do, but from the fermentation of sugar. Oxygen is dethroned in cancer cells and replaced by an energy-yielding reaction of the lowest forms, namely, a fermentation of glucose. Rapid reproduction of the cancer cells uses up large amounts of glucose, breaking it down into lactic acid. Lactic acid is a waste product that puts a strain on the body and causes an imbalance in the acid/alkaline ratio, or pH. As the acidity of the body rises it becomes even more difficult for the cells to use oxygen normally.

As cancer cells begin to multiply, forming a tumor, the liver must expend a considerable amount of energy converting the toxic lactic acid back to glucose. Also, most cancer cells can function only at a low pH (a very acidic state) because of the lactic acid they constantly produce. The combined effect of the tumor's metabolism is to tax the liver and acidify the body. Cancerous tumors may contain as much as ten times more lactic acid than healthy tissues. Remember, cancer cells *cannot* exist in an oxygen-rich environment!

An acid condition in the body can cause cells to become malignant. The acidity the intracellular fluids within the cell damages the cell nuclei which control cellular growth. Acidity in the extra cellular fluids kills the nerve cells that are connected with the brain reducing its ability to send proper messages to fight the dysfunctional cells (cancer). Alkalized water's micro clusters, which are made up of five to six water molecules, as a result of the electrolysis process, are able to effectively enter the cells and remove the acid thus increasing the body's ability to fight the free-radicals.

*"Of all the knowledge, the one most worth having is knowledge about health! The first requisite of a good life is to be a healthy person."*

Herbert Spencer

## So, What's in Your Water?

If we want to have safe drinking water and also avoid the potentially harmful effects of inhaling water pollutants or absorbing them through our skin, a first step is to understand the kinds of pollutants that may be in our water. Nuisance pollutants are those that cause discomfort or inconvenience. They can cause water to taste, smell, or look bad, and they can render soap and washing less effective. The following are health-threatening pollutants:

- Pathogens
- Toxic minerals and metals
- Organic chemicals
- Radioactive substances
- Additives

# Pathogens

Pathogens are harmful microorganisms such as bacteria, viruses and parasites. They can cause such diseases as typhoid, cholera, hepatitis, flu, and giardiasis. The most common bacteria are closely monitored in public water supplies. Private wells may be contaminated with bacteria. If the well is near a septic system, open to the air, or subject to chemical pollution or animal fecal matter.

Viruses are much smaller than bacteria and harder to detect. Viruses are very common in water. Although disinfected with chlorine (the method used by most public utilities) probably kills the majority of viruses in the water, no one knows for sure how many viruses remain potent.

The third type of pathogens commonly found in water is protozoan parasites. In people that have a suppressed immune system, these can be life threatening. Parasites can be present in public water supplies even though a water treatment plant is operating properly.

## Toxic minerals

Toxic minerals are the harmful *inorganic* substances that are found in water supplies. They include metals as well as common minerals in the form of rock, sand, and clay. The *inorganic* minerals in water that are known to be harmful to our health in large quantities are:

Aluminum

Arsenic

Asbestos

Barium

Cadmium

Chromium

Copper

Fluoride

Lead

Mercury

Nitrate

Selenium

Silver

Nitrite

These toxic minerals and inorganic compounds occur naturally in water, and they also enter water from man-made sources. Some of them are more toxic than others. Cadmium, lead, and mercury have the greatest toxicity, and ingestion of even small amounts can be fatal. Asbestos is also present in tap water wherever asbestos-cement water pipes are used to deliver water to customers. Trace-minerals are *organic* absorbable and found in plants, algae and some supplements. These (chromium, copper, silver) are safe and beneficial to the body in the proper dosage. Inorganic minerals cannot be absorbed by the body, resulting in toxicity.

## Organic Chemicals

Organic chemicals are substances that come directly from, or are manufactured from, plant or animal matter. Plastics, for example, are organic chemicals that are made from petroleum, which originally came from plant and animal matter. There are over 100,000 different manufactured, or synthetic, organic chemicals in commercial use today. In addition to the organic chemicals that have found their way into water supplies. New and dangerous one are created in the process of water treatment. Chlorine, which is added to essentially all U.S. public supplies, combines with organic compounds from decaying plant matter or sludge found in water system pipes, to form a category of toxic pollutants called trihalomethanes (THMs) that are carcinogens (substances that increase the risk of getting cancer).

# Radioactive Substances

Radioactive substances in water fall into two categories: radioactive minerals and radioactive gases. Radioactive minerals can be either naturally occurring or man-made. When naturally occurring, their source is typically an area where mining is going on or has gone on in the past. Uranium mining produces radioactive runoff. There are other kinds of mines that enable radioactive minerals to enter water supplies. This is because mining exposes rock strata, most of which contain some amount of radioactive ore. Naturally occurring radioactive minerals also can enter water supplies through the operation of smelters and coal-fired electrical plants.

Man-made sources of radioactive minerals in the water are nuclear power plants, nuclear weapons facilities, radioactive materials disposal sites, and docks for nuclear-powered ships. Another source of radioactive pollution comes from hospitals all over the country, which are allowed to dump low-level radioactive wastes into sewers. Some of those radioactive wastes eventually find their way into water supplies.

## Additives

Most public water treatment plants, from small community systems to larger urban waterworks, add things to water. These are added for a variety of reasons, ranging from disinfection to enhancing effectiveness of treatment to improving the water's aesthetic qualities.

The best-known additive is chlorine as mentioned earlier. According to studies conducted jointly at Harvard University and the Medical College of Wisconsin, the consumption of chlorinated drinking water accounts for 15 percent of all rectal cancers and 9 percent of all bladder cancers in the U.S. Further, people drinking chlorinated water over long periods of time have a 39 percent increase in their chances of contracting rectal cancer and a 21 percent increase in the risk of contracting bladder cancer.

## Water fluoridation

Fluoride, a poison second in toxicity only to arsenic, has routinely been added to public drinking water and toothpaste since the 1950s, despite mounting evidence of its health hazards. According to the scientific research, fluoride consumption creates multiple hazards with respect to cancer. Fluoride can actually produce cancer, transforming normal human cells into cancerous ones, even at concentrations of only 1 ppm (parts per million), the official "safe" dosage set by the U.S. Public Health Service for drinking water.

**Flocculants**

In addition to chlorine, and sometimes fluorine (a component of fluoride), water treatment plants often add several other substances to water to improve the efficiency of the treatment. Flocculants are substances added to water to make the particles in it clump together for more efficient removal by filtering.

Some of the most commonly used flocculants, called polyelectrolytes, have been banned in several other countries because some of their constituents are known to cause genetic mutations. The EPA classifies some of these flocculants as probable human carcinogens.

*"Only I can change my life. No one else can do it for me."*

Carol Burnett

# Sports Drinks and Bottled Water

Recently, there has been introduced to the market, a flurry of sport drinks, mixes, and electrolyte supplements. The marketing goals appear to be focused on rehydration and increased sports performance. Certain preservatives, artificial flavors and colored dyes, aspartame, and sugar may add to the visual or taste appeal of the drink, but may not be user-friendly to the body.

While most companies producing the products seem to embrace the value of electrolytes, they may not have delivered the proper complement of trace-minerals for formation and absorption. For example, Boron is a necessary trace element needed for cellular absorption of other nutrients. Since most sports drinks contain only sodium and potassium rather than the proper complement of multi-minerals, they are unable to create the proper reaction to make electrolytes that are needed to keep the body's electrical system charged.

In addition to its usefulness after exercise to replenish glycogen stores, sugar (fructose, dextrose, glucose, high fructose corn syrup, maltodextrin) is usually added as a carbohydrate to boost energy levels. While this may stimulate the body momentarily, minutes later the glycemic roller coaster sets in with associated compromise in body function.

Different studies reveal that sugar actually diffuses the body's ability to maintain muscle strength; therefore, it does not seem wise to use it when periods of strength are required. Sugar also creates cravings that generate a desire for more sweet drinks. In high quantities it also has been linked to diabetes. As blood glucose levels increase, people with diabetes are more at risk for heart disease.

Besides sugared drinks, there are other ways to get carbohydrates, such as energy bars, and the complex carbohydrates found in apples, grapes, or peanuts. Furthermore, studies show that it may be the complex carbohydrates that support strength and endurance, rather than simple carbohydrates. As for other aspects of water, there can be a wide variation in the quality of bottled water from one type or brand to another.

Among the many weaknesses of the FDA (Food and Drug Administration) regulation is the fact that the FDA exempts intrastate bottled water (bottled water not sold outside the state where it originates) from regulation, even though 75 percent of all bottled water sold in the United States is intrastate. Seltzer, other carbonated waters, and flavored waters are also exempted. The FDA requires testing of bottled water less frequently than is required by the EPA (Environmental Protection Agency) for tap water and if a particular bottled water exceeds the limits for any pollutants, that water can still be legally sold.

## Plastic Water Bottles

When water is placed in soft plastic bottles, it tends to leach out any chemicals in the plastic that are loosely bonded. These chemicals then enter the water in miniscule amounts. The longer water remains in a plastic bottle and the higher its temperature, the greater the chance of chemicals entering the water. For example, leaving a plastic water bottle in the car during the warm weather (and as the temperature rises in the car), the chemicals from the plastic bottle leach into the water, especially if you reuse these bottles. Most plastic bottles are for one-time use. No guarantees are made for the integrity of the chemical bonding for multiple uses.

Some studies have shown a link between chemicals leached from plastic water bottles and disorders of the immune system. Recently the FDA has been asked to review the safety of food products that contain bisphenol-A, or BPA, a hormone-disrupting chemical most commonly used in the linings of polycarbonate water bottles, specifically those marked with a #7 inside the recycled symbol on the bottom of the container. We highly recommend consumers use either glass or stainless steel bottles. This also helps to reduce landfill waste.

Electrolyte products are available to put in the refillable water bottles so you can make your own sports drink and control your intake of sugars. According to Nina Anderson, SPN, "sweetened sports drinks contribute to the obesity epidemic in the USA. Most of them also contain only sodium and potassium, which do not make effective electrolytes. We need in addition trace amounts of selenium, boron, copper, manganese, zinc, cobalt, silica, iodine and chromium to properly rehydrate the body."

*"Seek not to learn, but to think. Seek not to accept what is told to you, but to question."*

Bernard Jensen, D.C., Ph.D.

# The Amazing Benefits of Drinking Alkalized Water

From the moment of birth, our bodies are subjected to stress. We are assaulted by chemicals and pollutants in the atmosphere, the substances in our food, and by energetically harmful frequencies in the home and workplace. Each of these can cause excessive acidic waste and free radical damage resulting in sickness and premature aging!

The water we drink plays a major role in exacerbating or reducing the effects of these factors. Because our bodies are mostly water, this life-sustaining fluid is involved in all of our biological functions. Water has a major impact both on the aging process and on our body's ability to function optimally. That is why it is critically important to understand the difference between "dead water" and *alkalized water.*

There are many benefits to drinking alkalized water. The most important feature of alkaline water produced by a water ionizer is its Oxidation Reduction Potential (ORP). Water with a high Negative ORP is of particular value in its ability to neutralize oxygen free radicals. The negative ions in alkaline water from an electrolysis machine are a rich source of electrons that can be donated to these free radicals in the body, neutralizing them and stopping them from damaging healthy tissues. ORP is a measure of antioxidant power and is measured in millivolts (mV). It measures the presence of free electrons. A negative ORP means that a substance can donate free electrons, making it an antioxidant. A positive ORP means that a substance is taking electrons, making it a free radical or pro-oxidant.

Oxidation occurs when the oxygen molecule loses its electron and it becomes a free radical that begins to search for any molecule that might have an extra electron. Oxidation is how our bodies age resulting in wrinkles, degeneration of organs, bones, muscles, tendons, and cellular membranes. A reducing agent is simply something that inhibits or slows the process of oxidation.

The ORP of most tap water in the USA is between +200 to +600mV and so is an oxidizing agent. High pH ionized water demonstrates a negative (-) ORP and so is a reducing agent or "antioxidant". Most bottled waters are very acidic (low pH) and also have higher ORP's (over +400mV).

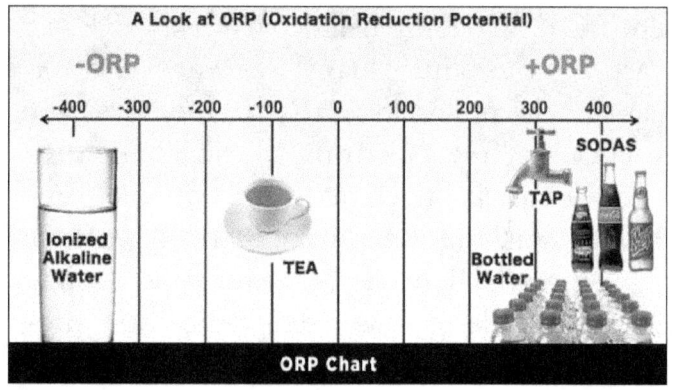

All water does not help hydrate the body efficiently. Distilled water is dead water and devoid of all minerals. It is very acidic and will tend to dehydrate us. Almost all distilled water has a pH of 4.5, that means this water is 1000 times more acidic than our blood which is pH 7.35. Reverse Osmosis water has many of the same problems. R/O water averages around a pH of 5, 100 times more acidic than our blood.

What most people don't know is that if our (tissue) pH drops below 5.8 we are not able to absorb vitamins A, B, E, F and zinc, no matter how much of these vitamins we take. Majority of people have a urine pH below 5.8 (normal 6.4) and don't realize that they are wasting their money on supplements.

Restructured alkaline water is the fastest and most efficient way to alkalize our body. The pH level of our internal fluids affects every cell in our body. Extended acid imbalances of any kind are not well tolerated. The entire metabolic process depends on a balanced internal alkaline environment. The most powerful program to reduce or eliminate these effects is to remove acid from the blood and tissues with an alkaline lifestyle and wise dietary and water consumption choices.

Another amazing benefit of drinking ionized alkaline water is that it assists in the absorption of minerals and other nutrients.

Especially when adding Cellular PSP. The combination of alkalized water and Cellular PSP together, increases the absorption rate, keeps our cells healthy and creates more energy.

> *"I learned to listen to my body with an inner concentration like meditation, to get guidance as when to exercise and when to rest learned that healing and cure are active processes in which I myself needed to participate."*

Rollo May

# Polysaccharides and Polypeptides (PSP)

Scientists have utilized ancient Thai folk medicine, techniques, and theory, combined with modern and sophisticated technology to produce polysaccharide peptides ("polysaccharidepeptides) or PSP. Alphaglycanology is a proprietary and innovative process employing biotechnology and nanotechnology. The purpose of the Alphaglycanology technique is to mechanically hydrolyze polysaccharides (complex carbs) and polypeptides (amino acids) in cereal grains, from specially selected fractions of rice grains, harvested at the proper age. The grain is grown in an area where the soils are alkaline in nature and continuously enriched with natural organic matter containing abundant spirulina found in the water. The rice is organically grown, free of pesticides and insecticides and is not modified in any way.

By bonding the polysaccharide peptides together under controlled humidity, temperature and pressure, a naturally hydrolyzed alpha-glycan is formed. Therefore, when PSP enters the body, the cells can recognize it as a biological fuel for utilization by the mitochondria for the production of the cellular energy or *ATP* (adenosine triphosphate).

The special characteristics of PSP produced with the Alphaglycanology process, allows for 100 percent bioavailability. When consumed, these unique functional genomic nutrients are readily assimilated facilitating an improvement of the intracellular environment. This is essential for DNA repair and the resulting enhanced gene expression. Correspondingly, the environment manifested in the body is vitally essential for optimal health. The Alphaglycanology process employed by scientists to produce PSP has shown its ability to effectively preserve the functional value of the phytonutrients.

Scientists have found that when certain species of rice grains are grown under optimal conditions, and are harvested at the proper age, they contain top quality functional and essential nutrients such as specific polysaccharides, polypeptides, the amino acids, vitamins, minerals, and antioxidants (gamma oryzanol, tocopherol tocotrienols). Rice grains meeting these criteria are perfectly suited to enhance the cellular energy (ATP) production of the mitochondria for DNA repair and cellular regeneration. They can combat free radicals and enhance the detoxification process establishing an anabolic (building) phase so that the body's natural healing power may function optimally. The unique combination of these antioxidants, organic mineral amino acid compounds, and polysaccharides, has the ability to stimulate the body to naturally regulate a state of *homeostasis* (when the body is in balance). This results in balanced levels of blood sugar, cholesterol, triglycerides, blood pressure, body temperature, electrolytes, and pH.

## Detoxification

An important function of PSP is its ability to detoxify the body. Avoiding contact with toxins on a daily basis is virtually impossible, and a buildup of these toxins within the body results in many forms of illness.

Cleanliness, externally and internally, is essential to good health. PSP assists this process because it works on the entire body to remove toxins from the system. When these toxins are eliminated PSP helps support and strengthen the glandular system helping the body heal itself.

The colon and the bowel become the depository for all waste material after food nutrients are extracted into the bloodstream. Decaying food ferments and forms gases as well as second and even third generation toxins. Thus the colon becomes a breeding ground for putrefactive bacteria, viruses, parasites, yeast and more. Because of PSP's fiber-like structure the peristalsis movement of the colon is strengthened and bowel movements are healthier and more regular, better facilitating the elimination process. Healthy intestines are the body's second immune system. Therefore, it is essential to keep them free of putrefied waste.

*"Treatment originates outside you;*
*healing comes from within."*

Andrew Weil M.D.

# *Fountain of Youth*

Through my research I have determined that PSP can play a big role in our search for the "fountain of youth." The antioxidant properties of PSP prevent body components from destruction by free radicals—a key to anti-aging.

The three important contributors to aging are: cell and tissue damage caused by free radicals; reduced immune response, and enzyme depletion in the body due to diets composed of enzyme deficient foods (cooked or processed.)

Free radicals, (highly active compounds produced when molecules react with oxygen,) play a key role in the deterioration of the body. Under assault from chemicalized foods and environmental pollutants, our bodies generate excesses of these cell damagers. After years of free-radical assaults cells become irreplaceably lost from major organs such as the lungs, liver, kidneys, the brain, and particularly our nervous system. This loss is seen as a primary cause of aging.

Alzheimer's, Parkinson's, and Multiple Sclerosis are thought to be associated with the aging process due to three potent neurotoxins, Beta-Amyloid, Glutamate, and Peroxides, that can lead to nerve cell damage and destruction. These molecules disrupt and destroy normal nerve cell function.

Studies reveal that PSP has been shown to preserve nerve cell function by supplying food and nutrients at the cellular level. The concept is simple. Provide the cell with food easily recognized and utilized by the cell's DNA (the "molecule of life") to generate energy. This will provide the vehicle for repairing cell damage.

This is incredible news for people with Alzheimer's and Creutzfeldt-Jakob diseases. Both illnesses manifest when a neurotoxin, called Beta Amyloid, deposits itself in the brain and disrupts communication between nerve cells. Scientists have tried to treat the diseases by attacking the protein deposits but to date this approach has not been successful.

A new study shows that by helping nerve cells produce normal proteins these connections can actually be rejuvenated. In this study, nerve cells exposed to three of the most potent neurotoxins were ultimately protected from damage after adding PSP to the medium. A degree of cellular regeneration of the nerve dendrites and axons was also seen. These extraordinary results have consistently been observed in subsequent research.

Superoxide dismutase (SOD) is an extremely potent antioxidant enzyme that fights cellular damage from single oxygen molecules (also known as free radicals). As an enzyme, SOD has particular value helping to protect against cell destruction. Research suggests that SOD may be the most important enzyme in the body for the control of free radicals, keeping our cell membranes young, supple, and healthy (anti-aging). Although SOD has been sold as a supplement, research shows that oral SOD is destroyed by the digestive system before it can fight free radicals and repair damaged joints. This suggests that the most viable means of building healthy levels of

SOD in the body would be to consume natural food substances that bind protein to SOD and therefore deliver it via the digestive system to the body, without being destroyed in the gut. PSP facilitates that process and increases the level of SOD in the body.

There are numerous antioxidants made by the body as well as antioxidants found through supplementation or in our diets. Nutrients like vitamins E and C, beta-carotene and the trace mineral selenium root out any free radicals that make it past the antioxidants enzymes. It is necessary to support the body's own production of antioxidant enzymes (SOD) because they remove free radicals three to ten times faster than the nutrient antioxidants. The body will benefit far more if it can produce its own antioxidant enzymes, and that is what PSP facilitates.

PSP is a premier agent for reversing the causes of aging by utilizing the following:

1. Increasing the level of SOD; (superoxide dismutase), the master antioxidant;

2. Enhancing nucleotide production for DNA repair;

3. Enhancing cellular environment for improved genetic expression;

4. Increasing pro-enzyme and probiotic (friendly intestinal bacteria) activities.

*"It is easy to get a thousand prescriptions but hard to get one single remedy."*

Chinese proverb

# Cellular Nutrition

Our bodies are confronted daily by excessive production of free radicals caused by our polluted environment, stressful lifestyles, and over-medicated society. Though we can certainly reduce the amount of free radicals our bodies' produce (not smoking, decreasing stress levels, and avoiding toxic chemicals), our bodies are still unable to fight the overwhelming daily attack on the natural defense system.

Since the last century, nutritional medicine and supplementation has focused on replenishing nutritional deficiency. Countless hours and dollars have been spent trying to determine exactly which nutrients our bodies have depleted. Blood tests, urine tests, hair samples, and muscle testing have been conducted in an attempt to determine which nutrients we need to supplement.

Mistakenly, we have been aiming at the wrong target. The present problem is not nutritional deficiency, but rather, underlying *oxidative stress*. Oxidative stress has now been shown beyond any shadow of a doubt via medical research, to be the root cause of over 72 chronic degenerative diseases. Diseases like heart disease, stroke, cancer, diabetes, arthritis, lupus, MS, etc.

Because oxidative stress is our concern rather than specific nutritional deficiencies, we must determine what is the best approach we should to take to help prevent or control oxidative stress. This can be accomplished by bolstering one's natural defenses through cellular nutrition.

Cellular nutrition is simply providing nutrients to the cell at optimal levels. This allows the cell to determine what it actually does and does not need. We really don't have to worry about determining which nutrients the cell is deficient in; we simply just provide the nutrients at optimal levels. Any nutritional deficiencies can be automatically corrected overtime by this approach and the other vital nutrients will be brought up to their optimal levels as well.

Cellular nutrition is providing the body with the antioxidants along with the supporting B vitamins and minerals at optimal levels. This is "preventative medicine" at its best because we can literally attack the disease process at its core by preventing oxidative stress from occurring.

Maybe you're wondering if we can control oxidative stress by simply improving our diet and eating more fruits and vegetables. This is definitely a good start. By simply eating 6 to 9 servings of organic fruits and vegetables each day, we can decrease the risk of heart attack, stroke, cancer, etc. We certainly want to supplement a good diet. Unfortunately, if we maintain a great diet we can barely obtain the RDA level of all essential nutrients. Numerous medical studies have shown that less than 1% of the American population accomplishes this on a consistent basis.

When the necessary nutrients (polysaccharides and polypeptides or PSP) are provided to the cell in a complete and balanced functional food, the combined effect is phenomenal. The potency of this food in optimizing our body's natural antioxidant, immune, and repair systems is maximized. Oxidative stress can be controlled and our health can be restored and protected.

Cellular nutrition is about health, not disease. Attacking the root cause of chronic degenerative disease is true preventative medicine. By applying these same principles, we who are in good health can decrease the risk of developing these chronic degenerative diseases.

# The Magic Within – The End to Old Looking Skin

Thin, old looking skin comes to us all, if we're lucky. However, when skin thins and ages prematurely, it can be depressing. There is no need to look old before our time. We can keep skin looking youthful for as long as possible if we treat it right. A healthy diet and avoiding skin damaging habits can go a long way in staving off old, thin looking skin.

Skin is the largest organ in the body, it primarily consists of two layers: the epidermis, which is the outer, visible layer of skin, and the dermis, which is a thick layer of tissue just beneath the epidermis. The dermis is responsible for supporting the epidermis. To that end, it is composed of a strong mesh of protein fibers, called collagen and elastin. These fibers play an essential role in the appearance of our skin. Collagen is responsible for skin's firmness, while elastin is responsible for skin's elasticity.

Skin starts to appear old when the body's production of collagen slows and the elastin fibers begin to lose their springiness. With the decreased production of collagen, the outer skin has less support and begins to sag. Further, because the elastin fibers have decreased elasticity, the skin does not "snap back" the way it used to, giving it a loose, aged appearance. To top it off, according to the American Academy of Dermatology, as we grow older, skin tends to lose its fat, making it thin-looking, and gravity pulls on it, making it droop.

Researchers have noted that changes to collagen and elastin begin in the mid-20s, although the subsequent changes in the skin don't usually become visible until decades later. However, some circumstances can hasten the weakening of these fibers, and make us look old before our time. Smoking and exposure to sun can damage collagen and elastin fibers, and greatly heighten the chances of developing wrinkles and sagging skin prematurely. In addition, other environmental factors, such as pollution and exposure to secondhand smoke, can also damage to skin fibers.

PSP also works to boost immune function in individuals in the following ways:

- Promotes healing skin cell renewal
- Assists in diminishing fine lines and wrinkles
- Refines and evens skin tone
- Helps combat free radical damage
- Improves skin resiliency, elasticity and firmness
- Helps tighten and cleanse skin
- Improves skin texture by enhancing cell structure
- 100% natural

*"The body is the soul's house. Shouldn't we therefore take care of our house so that it doesn't fall into ruin?*

Philo Judaeus

# Energy Drinks – Do We Really Need Them?

Energy drinks claim to provide people with increased energy levels that keep them active and alert. Energy drinks are sold in grocery stores, convenience stores, health food stores, bars, clubs, and in some areas, even schools. Are energy drinks safe and do we really need them?

Most energy drinks contain at least as much caffeine as a standard eight-ounce cup of coffee (80mg.). To put it into perspective, a 12oz. soda contains 18-48mg of caffeine. In addition to large doses of caffeine, energy drinks contain excessive amounts of sugar and legal herbal stimulants.

Children in school certainly do not need to be consuming any type of beverage that contains stimulants, particularly when they are

73

combined with sugar. Despite manufacturer claims to the contrary, marketing of energy drinks is targeted to high school kids, and adults who are under the 30years of age.

Many of us might already be aware of the basic contents mentioned above, however we still aren't exactly sure about the specific ingredients in energy drinks, and what effect those ingredients can have on our body.

**Common Energy Drink Ingredients:**

- **Ginseng** – A root that is believed to help reduce stress and increase energy levels.

- **Carnitine** – An amino acid that helps to metabolize fatty acids.

- **Gingko Biloba** – Created from the seeds of the gingko biloba tree, it has been shown to enhance memory.

- **Taurine** – A natural amino acid produced by the human body. Taurine helps to regulate normal heartbeats and muscle contractions. Its effect on people when consumed as a drink additive remains unclear.

- **Inositol** – A member of the B-complex vitamin that assists in the relaying of messages between cells. Inositol is not a vitamin itself.

- **Guarana Seed** – A stimulant that grows in Brazil and Venezuela, which contains high levels of caffeine.

Given this list of ingredients, it is fairly easy to see that energy drinks are a deceptive combination of soft drink and pseudo-nutritional supplement. The largest problem with them is that people tend to abuse them, drinking more than one at a time, or mixing with alcohol. There is becoming a high statistic of people being addicted to many of the energy drinks that are on the market today.

One of the main concerns with the use of herbs in these drinks is the source of these herbs. The manufacturers of energy drinks are not required by law to list whether or not the herbs they use have been sprayed with toxic pesticides, irradiated or watered with contaminated water, so there is no telling what toxins are contained in these drinks and whether or not these herbs will have negative effect on the body.

The caffeine that is found in energy drinks is dangerous enough on its own. Not only is caffeine addictive, it acts as both a stimulant and a diuretic. As a stimulant, excessive caffeine can lead to anxiety attacks, heart palpitations, and insomnia. Caffeine can also make us jittery or irritable. As a diuretic, caffeine causes our kidneys to remove extra fluid from our body. If we consume energy drinks while sweating, these effects can be particularly dangerous because we can become severely dehydrated quickly.

## What happens when energy drinks are combined with alcohol?

This combination carries a number of dangers:

- Since energy drinks are stimulants and alcohol is a depressant, the combination of effects may be dangerous. The stimulant effects can mask how intoxicated we are and prevent us from realizing how much alcohol we have consumed. Fatigue is one of the ways the body normally tells someone that they've had enough to drink.

- The stimulant effect can give the person the impression they aren't impaired. No matter how alert they feel, their blood alcohol concentration (BAC) is the same as it would be without the energy drink. Once the stimulant effect wears off, the depressant effects of the alcohol will remain and could cause vomiting in their sleep or respiratory depression.

- Both energy drinks and alcohol are very dehydrating (remember the caffeine in energy drinks is a diuretic). Dehydration can hinder our body's ability to metabolize alcohol and will increase the toxicity, and therefore the hangover, the next day.

PSP has been scientifically proven to increase cellular energy (ATP) production up to 54%. There isn't any "crash" or harmful side effects. PSP is regarded as the most unique functional food available. It can be readily assimilated and utilized by our body as food and works to provide the required energy at the cellular level (ATP) thus preventing the impairment of glucose/energy metabolism. It is anticipated to improve the ability of neurons to reduce the levels of free radicals and enhance the synthesis of ATP at the cellular level.

# Resources

Drinking fresh alkalized water gives the body more antioxidant power and deep hydration. Having a unit in your kitchen also makes it possible to drink as much pure alkalized water as your body desires every day with no waste of plastic bottles or concern about drinking plastic-contaminated water. The cost is considerably less over the life of the generator than bottles or designed water.

For further information, contact:

www.healthbesttoday.com

The polysaccharides and polypeptides in **Cellular PSP** (the original PSP) is the only natural functional food known to efficiently and effectively deliver a powerful combination of vital and essential nutrients to your body at the cellular level.

By including **Cellular PSP** in your daily diet, you provide your body's cells with exactly what they need to stay healthy!

For further information, contact:

www.healthbesttoday.com

*Let no one presume to give advice to others that has not first given good advice to himself.*

Seneca

## Conclusion

The information and statistics from the previous chapters will mean nothing to you unless you take action. This is more than a book about alkalized water and PSP. It is a book about people like you—individuals who are in search of health and natural healing. There are many people who feel that combination of drinking alkalized water and taking PSP have changed their lives. For some, it is miraculous, and for others it is significant enough to make the quality of their lives much better. You deserve the best quality of life, health, and wellness and drinking alkalized water and taking PSP can restore and preserve that health for a lifetime.

# About the Author

Dr. Howard Peiper is a Doctor of Naturopathic Medicine. In 1972, he received his degree in Naturopathy. After a decade in private practice, Dr. Peiper became a successful consultant, speaker and writer.

Throughout the years, his cutting edge articles appeared in numerous medical journals and magazines. He also serves on the medical advisory board for several nutritional companies.

Dr. Peiper has written several bestselling titles, including: *The A.D.D. and A.D.H.D. Diet*, *The Secrets to Staying Young* and *New Hope for Serious Diseases*. He is a frequent guest speaker on radio and television programs. He even hosted his own shows, including the award-winning television show, "Partners in Healing."

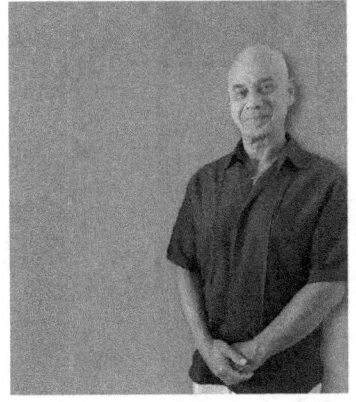